Combinatorial chemistry and multiple parallel synthesis

Afiya Ansari

Humeera Rafeeq

Ms. Tasleem

Contents

Combinatorial chemistry and multiple parallel synthesis 1

Definitions: 1

Introduction: 3

Solid-phase organic synthesis of informational macromolecules of interest to medical chemists 4

    Peptide arrays: 4

    Oligosaccharide arrays: 17

    Nucleoside Arrays: 18

    Lipid Arrays: 20

References: 23

PREFACE

The book is made by my own effort under the guidance of my lecturer that I have learned during my course. I have gained very precious knowledge by writing this book - Combinatorial chemistry and multiple parallel synthesis. Combinatorial Chemistry is emerging topic and has its wide applications in variety of fields. I have tried to put the best in this book.

Combinatorial chemistry and multiple parallel synthesis

Definitions:

Combinatorial chemistry is now having many different features which is merely tough to describe accurately. Basically parallel synthesizes assemblage of procedures that acknowledge the concurrent chemical synthesis of huge amount of compounds by using different ranges and varieties of reagents and initial materials. The total number of chemical compounds the definition covered chiefly begins at 25 members. The compound library obtained as a result can contain all the attainable chemical structures which can be synthesized by this procedure. Many scholars and scientists like better not to make use of the terminology combinatorial chemistry for procedures generating libraries that contain combination of compounds.

Multiple parallel synthesis is a connected association of methodologies used to synthesize a preferred minor, extended concenter and little assorted collection of compounds than those synthesized with combinatorial mechanizations. On a general basis parallel synthesis techniques synthesize library members as distinct compounds.

Solid-phase organic synthesis(SPOS) is in general terms accredit to the production of a target molecule in which the initial material is connected to a resin and stays through consecutive reagent analysis, usually till the end trial.

Phase trafficking occurs when a material or group of materials is relocated from one phase to another. This can involve relocation of liquid to liquid, liquid to solid transfers etc,.This methodology mergethe bonus of solution-phase organic synthesis and solid-phase organic synthesis.

Introduction:

Since past five years the chemical medicinal applications of combinatorial chemistry was revised in the particular succession. The field has developed considerably. Firstly the capability of making large chemical libraries having great informational macromolecules for conceptive screening determinations was quiet considerate and prominent. Currently this phenomenon has directed to other way with the cognizance that only a subset of the organic molecules which have the ability to produce has a genuine chance of developing to oral drugs. combinatorial chemistry emerged out of peptid3e chemistry accomplished on resin beads at first apportioned the essentials of biochemists and the subset of medicinal chemists who are specifically specialized in the particulars of peptide science. It is a fact that most people admit that the way preeminent to current scenario of combinatorial chemistry efficiently initialized with solid-phase synthetic experiments. The following work had instant force leading in great dimension as the reactions are characteristically constant and are compelled to the accomplishment with the use of reagents which are used in huge amounts are impressionable to automation and the debris can be evacuated from the products obtained by filtration or by basic washing. With the recent advance developments of screening techniques for drug discovery, the reserve work of presently extant artificial or natural molecules was processed through actualize a high appeal for new sources that chemists could surplus. The following need was accomplished by combinatorial chemistry. As very important injectable therapeutic agents, peptides, are metabolically very unstable for the production of splendid oral drugs. Benzodiazepine analogs was very firstly synthesized as potentially small oral drug like molecules by Bunin and Ellman in 1992 using resin bound solid phase organic synthesis techniques. This grabbed remarkable attention and now combinatorial chemistry and multiple parallel syntheses now spread throughout for all practical purpose at every branch of organic and medicinal chemistry. At first it was anticipated that the work of production of drugs like molecules with the help of combinatorial chemistry techniques would lead to the very quick production of many newer drugs as its result. This anticipation synchronized with the production of various potent targets for chemotherapy coming out of genetic engineering advances. This grew to the basic concern for the management branches to transfer the drug discovery criterion in pharma branches from the old traditional fashion to an industrial revolution approach.

Elemental chemical variety is more considerably far reaching than pharmacological adequacy and thus the hope for the advancement of development of new drugs failed to appear. To overcome these issue combinatorial techniques has been confined but today more importance is given to the synthesis of more genuine, smaller, compound libraries bearing drug like molecules with more efficacy.

The foremost advantage combinatorial chemistry and multiple parallel chemistryis high rate of the reaction for the synthesis of drug. Some compounds are produced within no time during synthesis of drugs, these compounds can be useful to medicinal chemist but these compounds cannot be specifically drugs. A huge amount of novel compounds are generated but the ratio of introduction of novel drugs into the market has been the same as before. An acknowledgement has been has been manifested to discern the varieties of typical features that molecules require in order to have a causative chance of becoming presentable orally active drugs. The work on combinatorial chemistry by Lipinski and Veber and coworkers principles are now general and are active as filters for molecules schemed for admittance in combinatorial libraries. Exhaustive work on knowing the structural obstruction is to acceptable absorption, distribution, metabolism and excretion characteristics. Side effects and toxicities are of major concern and optimistically will also be overthrown by excessive findings. When coupled with combinatorial chemistry techniques a novel start has been made in compound library design which will focus to the lead of wanted increase in useful productivity.combinatorial chemistry techniques now have more small, focused libraries that encourages for accomplishing libraries till the drug checking concern has reached its specific entity. In regard with various techniques, the productivity towards smaller, more focused compounds sets has taken away some applications of solid-phase chemical synthesis. Bead-based chemistry has also been evolved in a novel manner. Many reactions based on kinetics are solved by the use of solvent soluble and solvent insoluble polymers and also helped in productivity. Now-a-days phase trafficking has been efficiently and popularly used for elimination of unwanted by-products and excess or leftover reactants by the use of bead-bound reagents.

Everywhere now in industries and in academic laboratories use combinatorial techniques or methods as important source of their action and use them in a proper manner in drug searching. Maintenance of the shape of large legacy compound libraries having discrete compounds in millions for imitated sampling and screening, filling in dissimilarity gaps by aimed production, elimination of junk compound, determining identity, purity, stability, prevention of crashing out of solutions and undesirable molecular aggregation, regular checking of data, scrupulous betterment of individual compounds for formulation of screening sub libraries, its costs are still to be fully comprehend. Large number of companies have been emerged in account to provide specialized equipment's for the manufacturing process, mechanization, managing, separation processes and examination of combinatorial attempt. In defiance of a number of companies which have been developed for expansion of combinatorial chemistry and immense labor work, currently it is deemed that only one compound has made it all the way from initiation to FDA approval with the use of combinatorial chemistry.Sunitinib which is a vascular endothelial growth factor, platelet derived growth factor, tyrosine kinase inhibitor has been used in the treatment of renal cancer having advanced from High Throughput Screening (HTS) of combinatorial chemical compound library pursued by intensification and optimization of the originating hits.

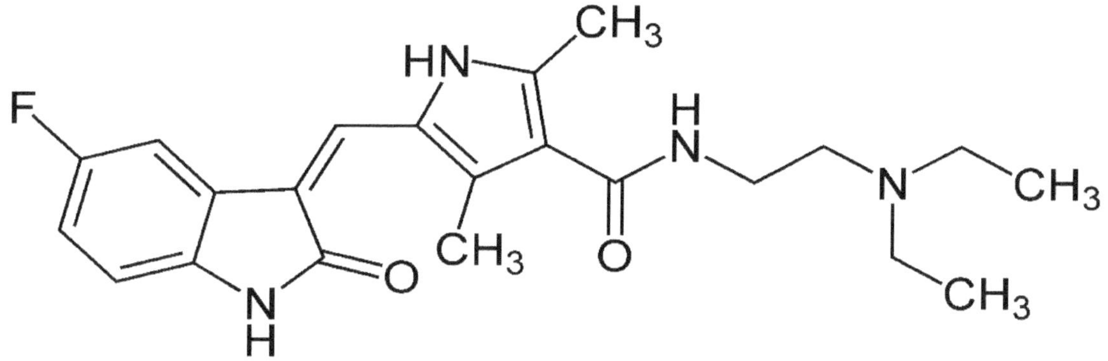

Fig1: The structure of Sunitinib.

Solid-phase organic synthesis of informational macromolecules of interest to medical chemists

Peptide arrays:

Peptide linkage has noteworthy benefits for combinatorial chemistry being stable chemically, nonchiral and constructible by constant series of operations manageable to automation. Peptides are exceptionally branched and it acquires a collection of remarkable biological properties and can be buildup with huge variety from readily accessible materials. Peptides are evident among the compounds of interest to biochemist. Peptide libraries are worthy in lead seeking in primary necessary studies on cellular operations, or for the manufacture of parenteral preparations for replacement therapies. Another aspect that can be noted in mind is that the manufacture of specific and definite medically valuable polypeptide drugs such as growth hormone and human insulin through genetic engineering operations is ably advanced and suitable or appropriate lessening the requirement for synthetic chemistry other than the manufacture of synthetic analogs. According to principles the value of peptides that can be synthesized in combinatorial mode is massive.

The easiest and less ambivalent method for establishing and deconvoltuting peptide libraries is dimensionally separate or spatially addressed method. For example a single polypeptide is manufactured on a unit type of resin and the products are kept separately. Decoding sequence is not required to be attached to the beads in this relative kind of library. The following method was put forth by Geysen in the year 1984 for the preparation of relevant array of peptide concurrently and to follow the products and promote their screening, the reactions were performed on resins attached to the ends of singular polyethylene pins so organized that they fix up into singular wells of microtiter plates.

A suitable deviation increasing the influence of split and mi libraries was introduced by R.A Houghten for parallel synthesis where in beads were comprised in porous polyethylene bags bathe into solutions of reagent and the following are termed as "tea bags". The unnatural operations employed a divide-couple-recombine design where singular residues were structured in the discrete bags which were distinctively isolated and so each individually could be tested without needing monotonous separation techniques. By this means the active sequences could be methodically acknowledged until the finest sequence became pure and clear. The individuality of the peptide or peptides confined is documented on the attached label. This opportune process incapacitated former confines by consenting the proclamation of products into solution so that they could interrelate with an extensive diversity of test systems. By the use of iterative synthesis and testing schemes, an orderly identification of the finest antigenic determinant was prepared from a chemical library of nearly 34 million hexapeptides. Scanning of the similar compound library also recognized antimicrobial peptides.

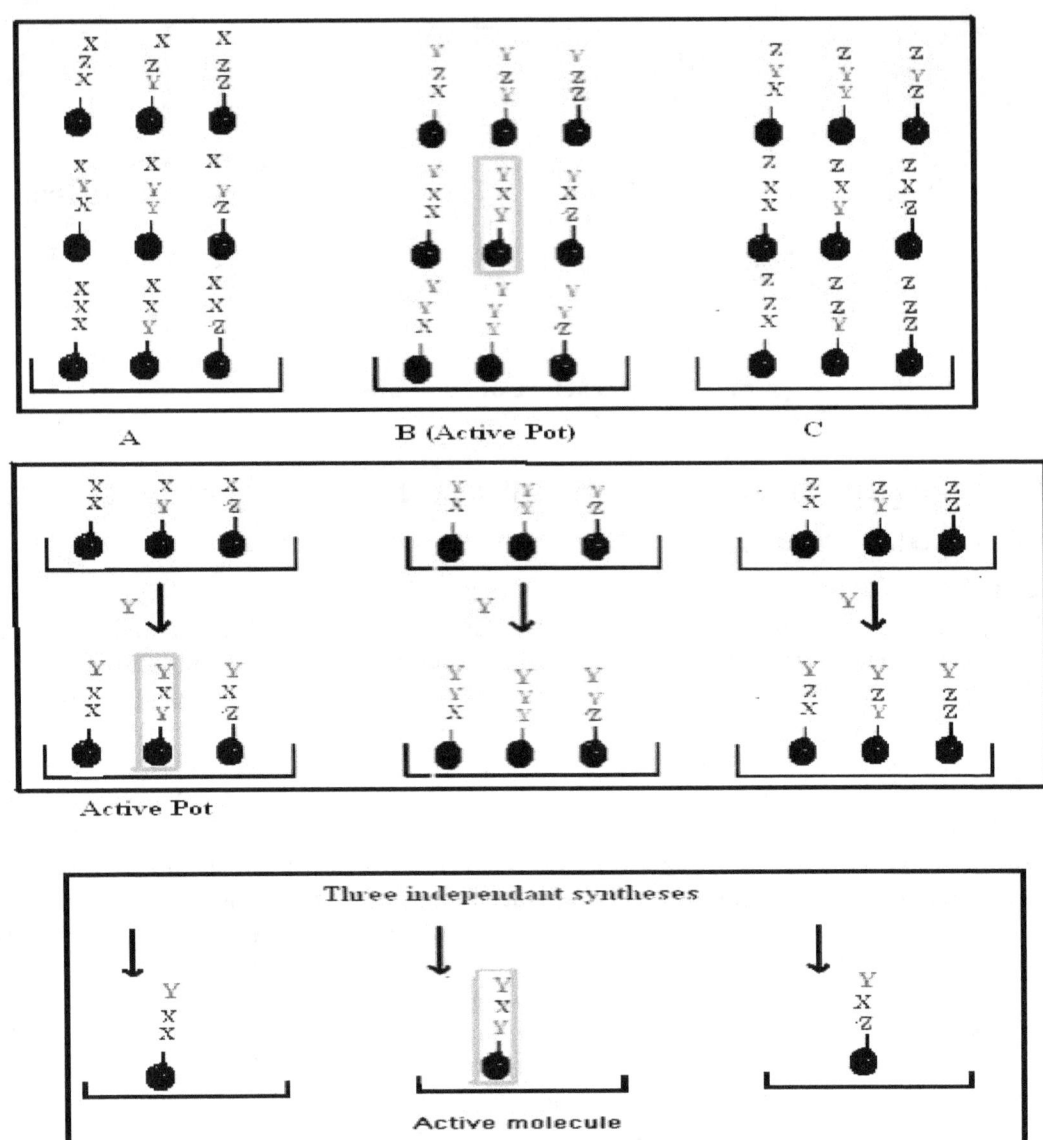

Fig2: The Houghton "Tea bag" method.

During the same period, Fodor technologically advanced an assorted library of 1024 peptides on silicon wafers with the use of photolithographic chemistry for protecting, forming, and releasing the peptides and also supervising the precise place along an axis where each peptide would be positioned through use of several configured masks. Photolytic protecting groups were hired followed by coupling the novel discovered "hot spots" with an appropriate reaction. The masks were often relocated by the following as preferred and the process is repeated. In standards, this procedure could produce thousands of individual peptides on a credit card like surface and is not restricted to peptides. This synthesis can be readily automated. Every library component dwells in a specific xy grid location. This method necessitates photosensitive protecting groups and testing methodologies well suited with support bound products.

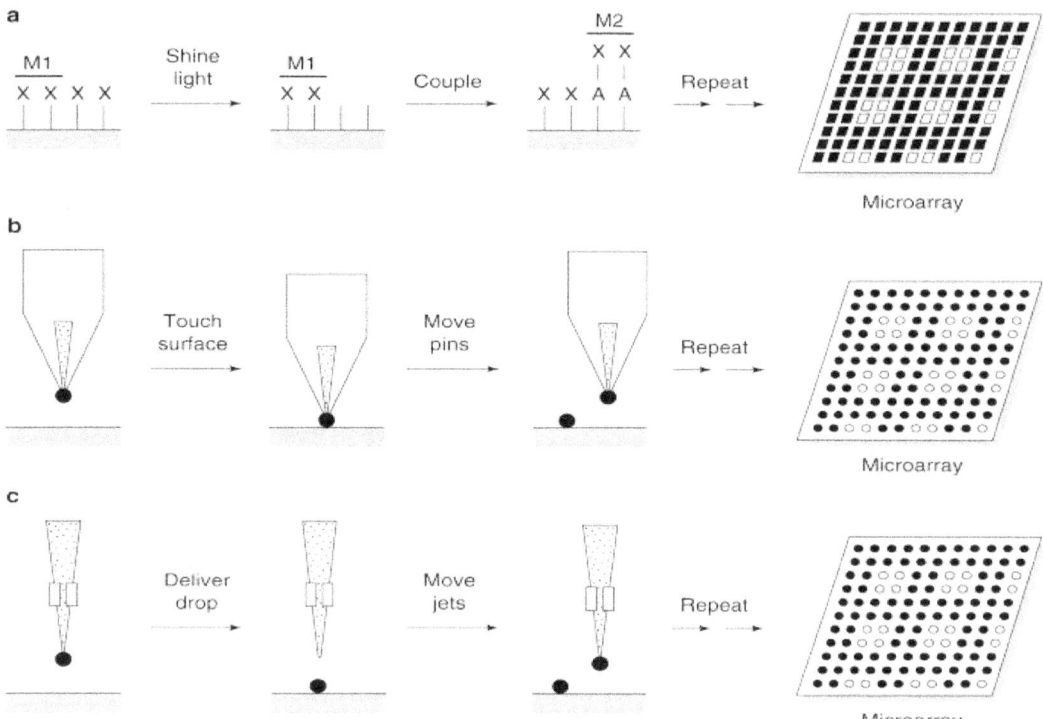

Fig3: Fodor photolithographic method.

An organic way that enables the making of huge arrays of peptides in solution has been progressed with the use of recombinant DNA techniques. Differrent kind of peptides are vented on the surface path of bacteriophages by introducing arbitrarily manufactured oligonucleotide sequences into the genome. Each and every resulting clones encodes for a different peptide. Natural amino acids only can be used in this method of synthesis. The active compound present are in suspension and the ligand is selected by the receptor by panning.

In the split and pool synthesis a first starting reaction is carried out on a bead support to attach an amino acid and the beads which are then produced are split into n number of equal portions and every single n group of beads are deprotected and is made to react with one of the group of second amino acids for the production of dipeptides and these are then deprotected and pooled again followed by thorough miing and finally the pool is further separated into equal proportions and these are then made to react with another group of amino acids for the production of group of tripeptide mixtures. The following succession of manufacturing operations is maintained constant until contented and the extreme group of resin piles is not mied frequently. Every single bead constitues of a single peptide but the end products with the help of this method comprises of groups of associated peptides all of which consisting of the same last amino acid if worked out in the organized sequencial manner. Lastly the beads are detached for testing purpose in the final step.

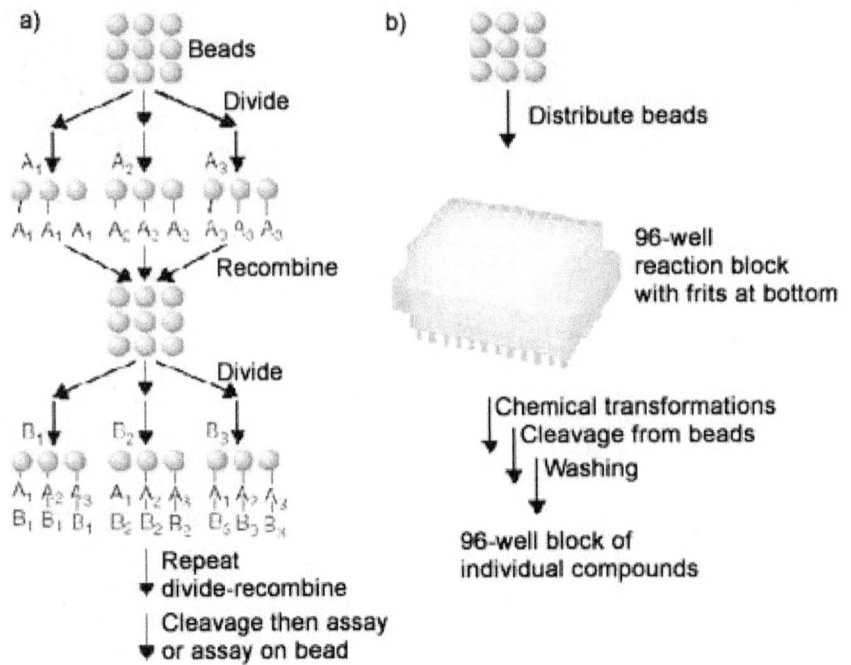

Fig4:The pool and split method.

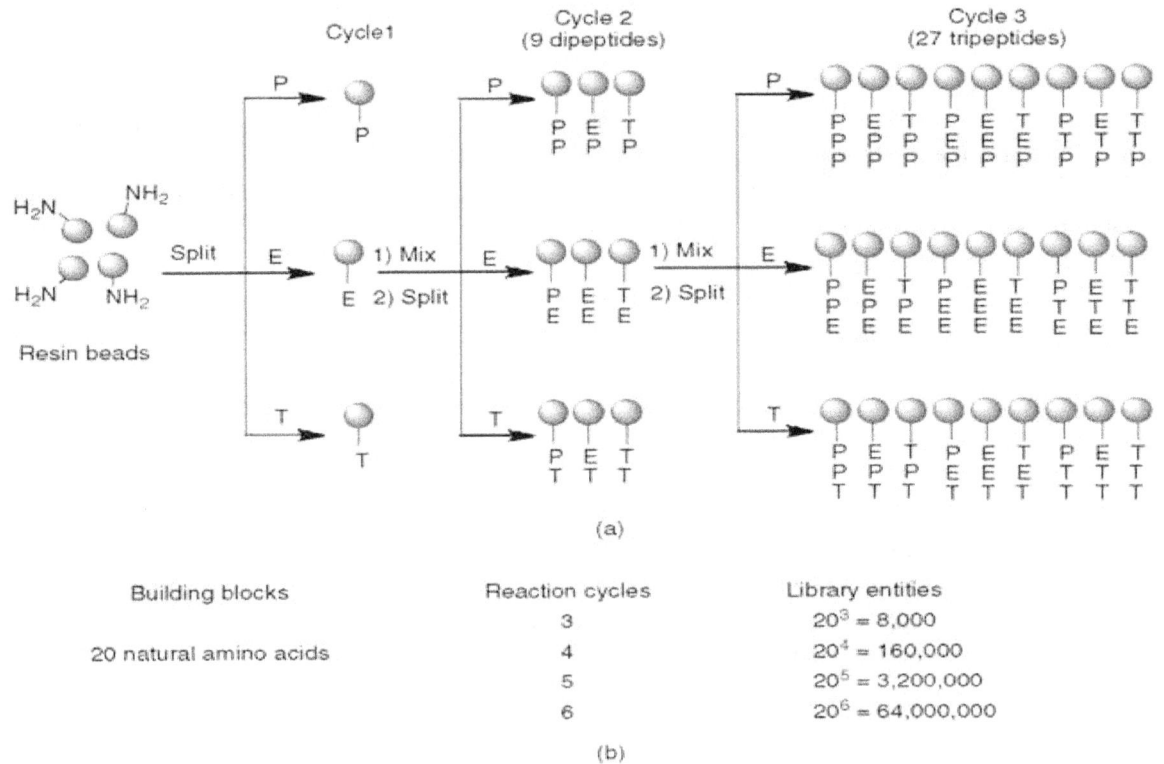

Building blocks	Reaction cycles	Library entities
	3	$20^3 = 8,000$
20 natural amino acids	4	$20^4 = 160,000$
	5	$20^5 = 3,200,000$
	6	$20^6 = 64,000,000$

(b)

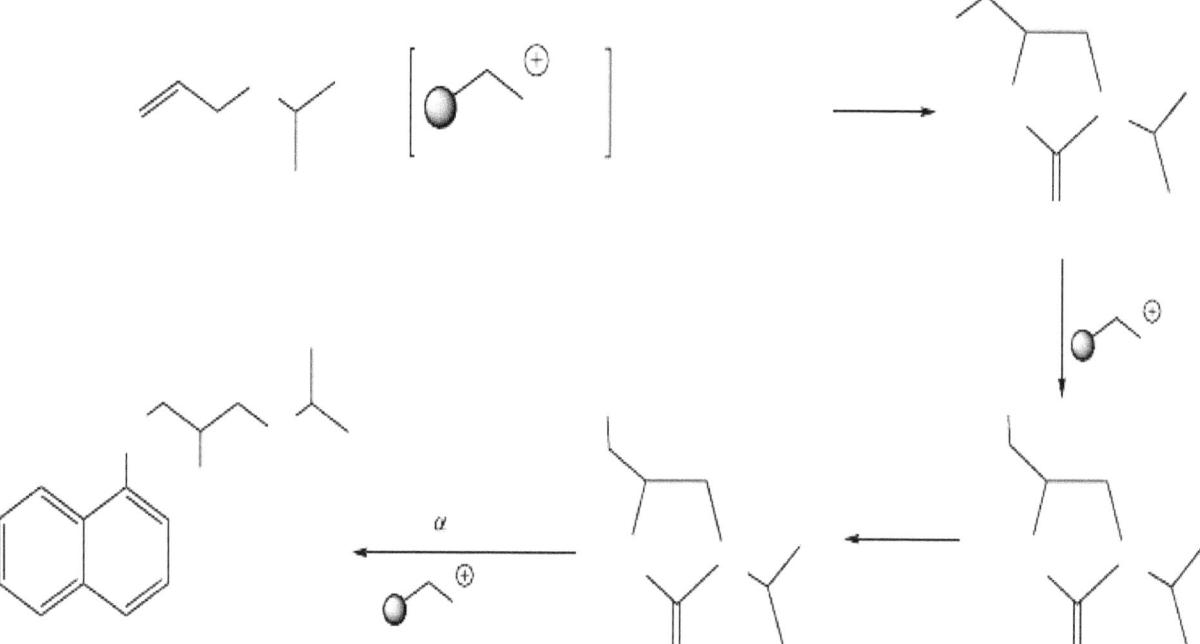

Fig5: Some eamples of the split and mix method with positional scanning.

A vast variety of peptides can be produced in many miture in small edict with the use of the above discussed methods. Numerous sub variations can be futher planned for future purposes. In common more than single peptide is obtained, making the repetition more multifaceted. The manufacture of all these active compounds as particular singular unadulterated chemicals will spontaneously lead to the elaboration of a structural activity relationship. The process is although strenouos, it has no prior conceptions and the remaining sequences which is not of much use can be omitted and inspected in future against various types of assays. One more advantage of the following method is that the final end products are not secured so are able to undertake the solution conformation verbalized by their sequence or by the receptor interactions and also interactions with the insoluble receptors.

In the omission or substitution method, individual omits individual of the amino acids form a certain specified position mostly from the end position. The following procedure is frequently repeated until all the activity is completely lost. By this procedure one can define the prime and optimum length of a peptide lead. Alanine scans encompass replacement of an amino acid residue at any preffered position by an alanine and determining the affect that is present in it which it has on bioactivity. The use of alanine helps to conserve the possible confirmation of the resulting analog. To determine the relative contribution of each amino acid side chain, this is method is applied at each position.

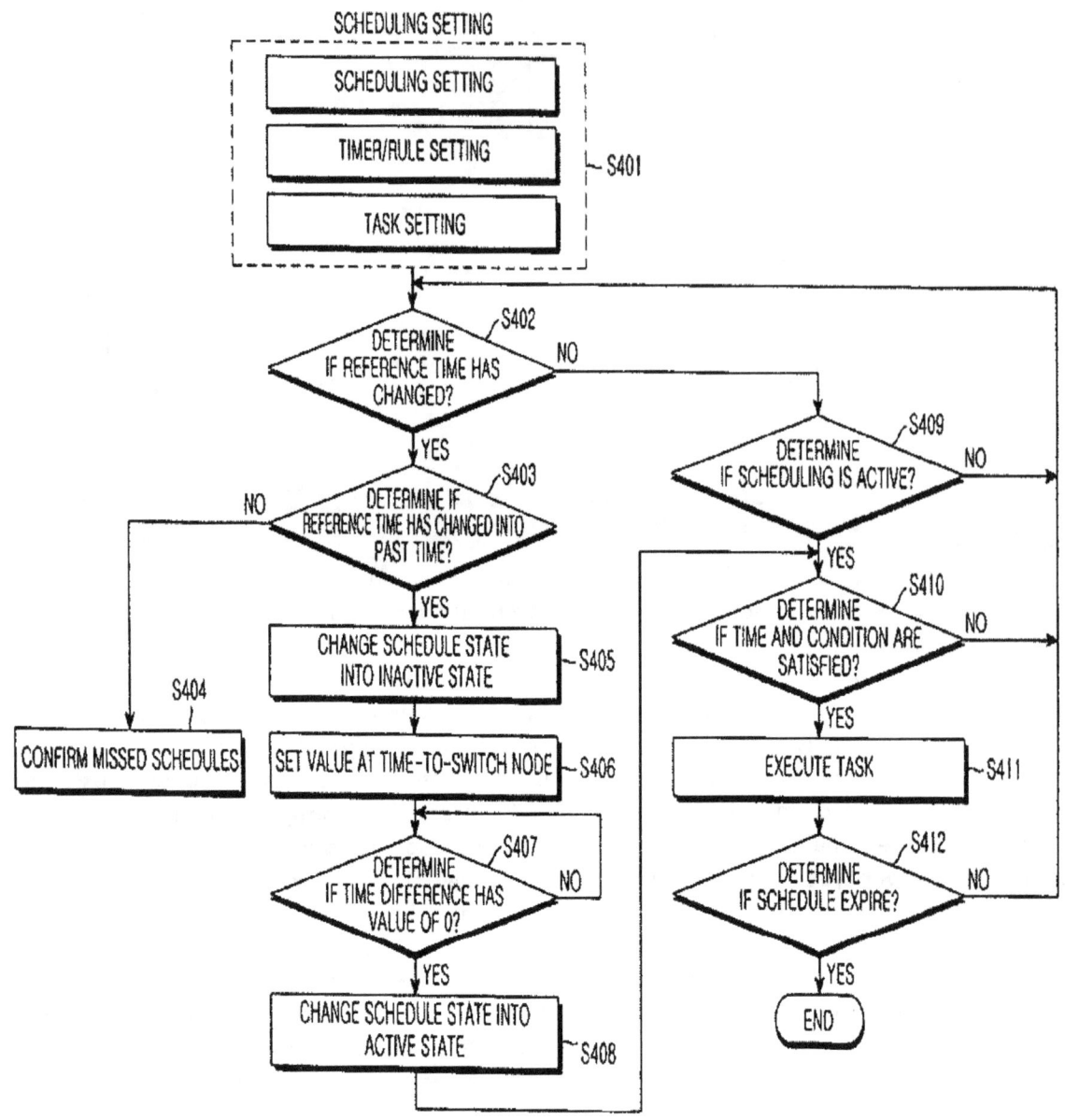

Fig6: The substitution/omission method.

Development by positional scanning is accelerated through testing groups of resins orderly arranged in checkerboard rows and columns. Consequent libraries are far tiner so that the procedure becomes gradually less laborious. Adding to the bioassay deconolutions, direct chemical procedures of sequence analysis are also existing. Mass spectroscopy is more famous for this as are NMR spectroscopy methods which involves magic angle methods on single beads. Also Edman degradation of peptides can be executed.

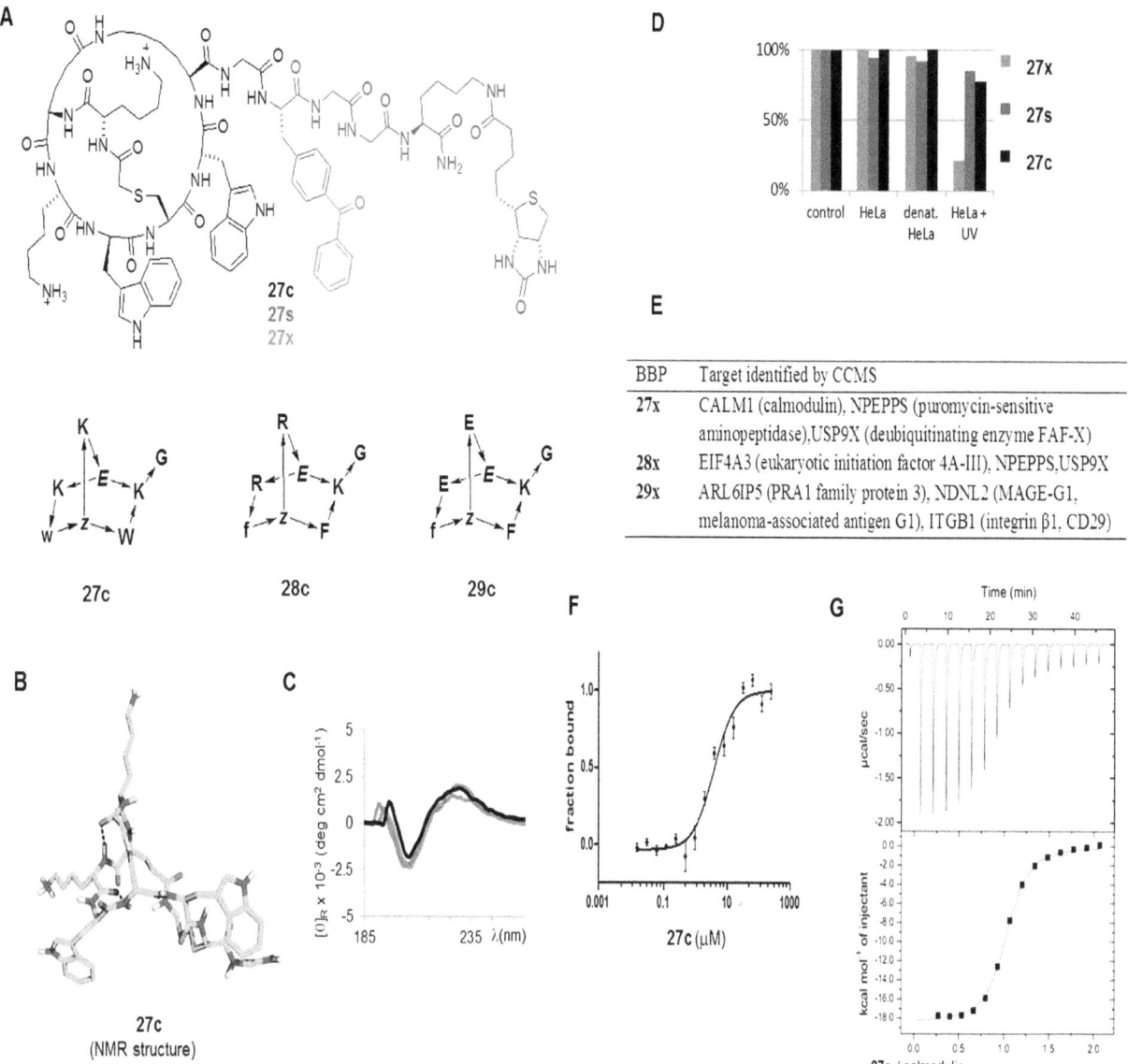

Fig7: Illustration of a resin with arms containing an analog and a signal sequence each of which can be removed independently from the resin.

An added well known method of recognizing definite residues of notice is to ascribe a non peptide signalling molecule to a separate arm. Every time a novel unit is added up like bonus to the new emerging and growing molecules. The coding and signalling molecules demands to be closely attached to its arm using chemistry that does not obstruct with the growing peptide on the other arm. There are many variable types of stratergies laboring in detaching the sequences from the arms. The active analogue needed to be decoded. The product which is emigrant before or after testing rests upon the necessities of the test protocol.

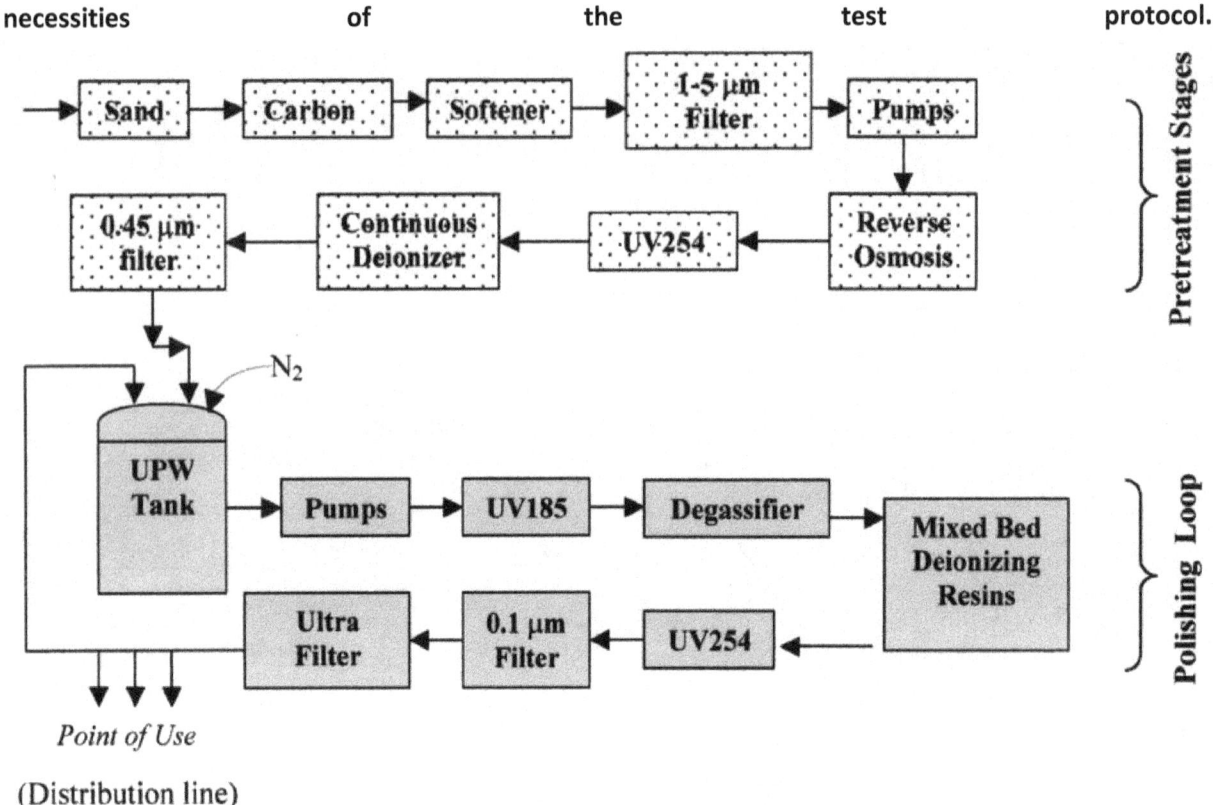

Fig8: some strategies for detachment of components and the products produced.

Detachment strategies signify an internal displacement reaction and leaves no traces behind in the product produced from the usual point of attachment. The signal sequence passes the antiquity of the bead and hence codes the antiquity of the sequence of steps implicated in the production and hence for the recognition of the peptide all of which are attached to the beads. The affluence of recognition or classification of oligonucleotide sequence by PCR methods has made is much more famous for such coding. Different types of halogenated aromatic residues have been used in the form of a binary code for the respective cause. Electron capture mass spectrometry is satisfactorily subtle to identify the codes on such beads. Encoding which uses adenylated secondary amines can also be performed. Stable isotopes can also be specifically used in precise ratios. Color coding along with the use of oil based organic dyes has also been used to a far extend to label single bead, single compound chemical libraries. These dyes are used in practice of application to the beads a little before testing for cell surface receptors. A further method is to set in an rf generator tuned to single frequencies in the resin itself so that the constituent present on the bead can be known by tuning to the accurate frequency. Substantial instrumental possessions are also obligatory in this method. By the use of combination of micro flow NMR and mass spectroscopy, decoding of individual peptides existing in 384 well microplate wells has also been performed. The split and mi peptide arrays can also be decoded by amino acid analysis of the materials on the beads by integrating an amino acid into two distinct positions in the sequence grouped in different pair liable on the length of the peptide. This has been verified and shown in compound library of 65,536 octapeptides although this is restricted to focus libraries.

Evidently with huge libraries it is precisely not conceivable to analyze each and every product so for this purpose another option instead of this method like statistical sampling should be operated so that each and every compound has been efficaciously synthesized.

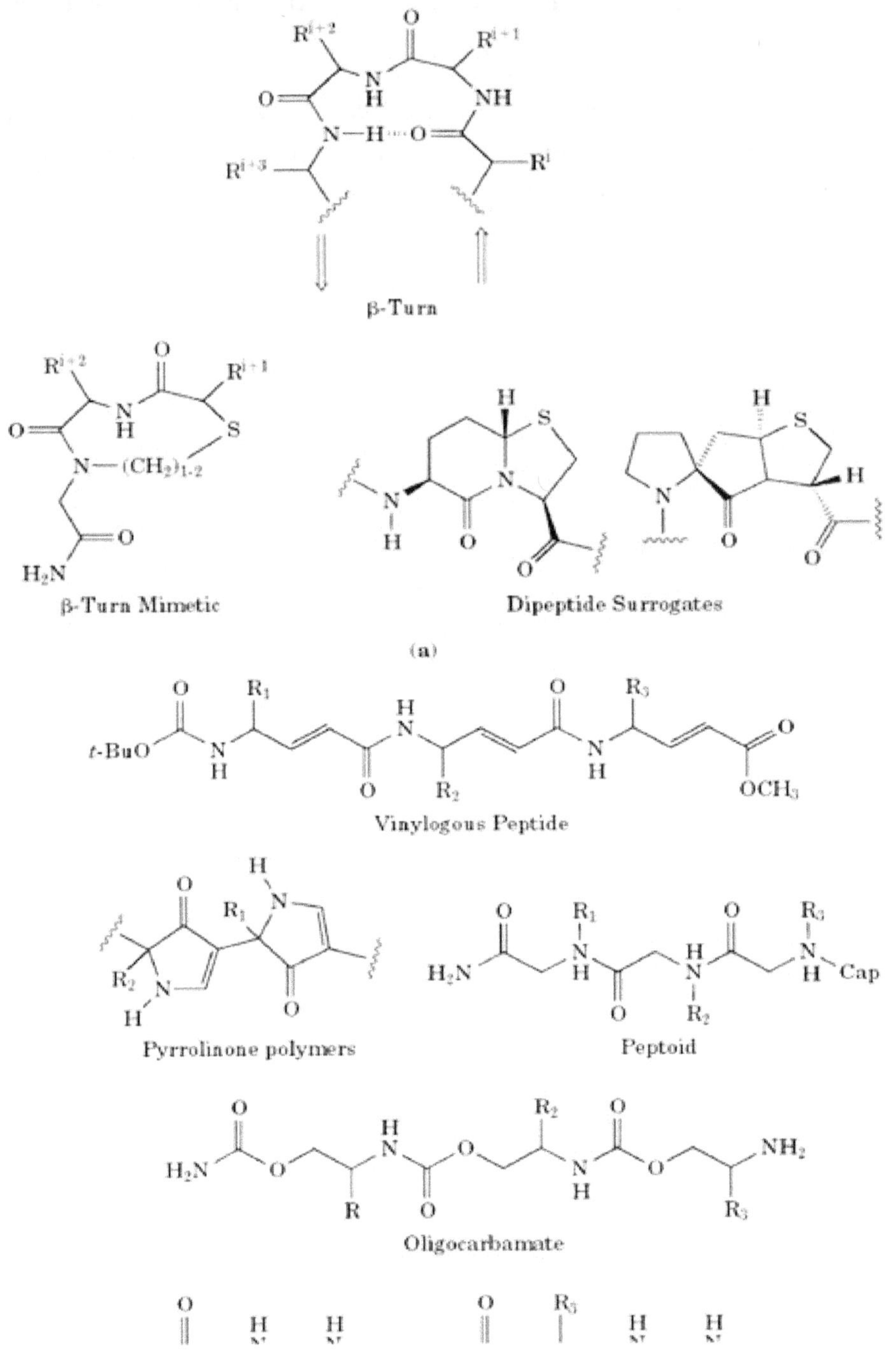

Fig9: some peptide surrogates employed in compound libraries.

With future advancement the peptide linkage began to alter itself and rework. For instance the conventional and standard style of stabilization against peptidase cleavage by transformation of the peptide bond NH into N-methyl consequently progressed into the synthesis of peptoids which are generally polygycine chains with every NH substituted with a variability of N-alkyl groups of the kind which will be similar to the side chains located in normal amino acids basically. Advancly the recent libraries have arisen where in the complete conformation of the peptide has been diversified by a heterocycle so that the resulting end product looks similar to topographically a beta turn. It is not necessary for the peptidomimetic group to merge any communal amino acid components. At present it is very energetic subject of medicinal chemistry.

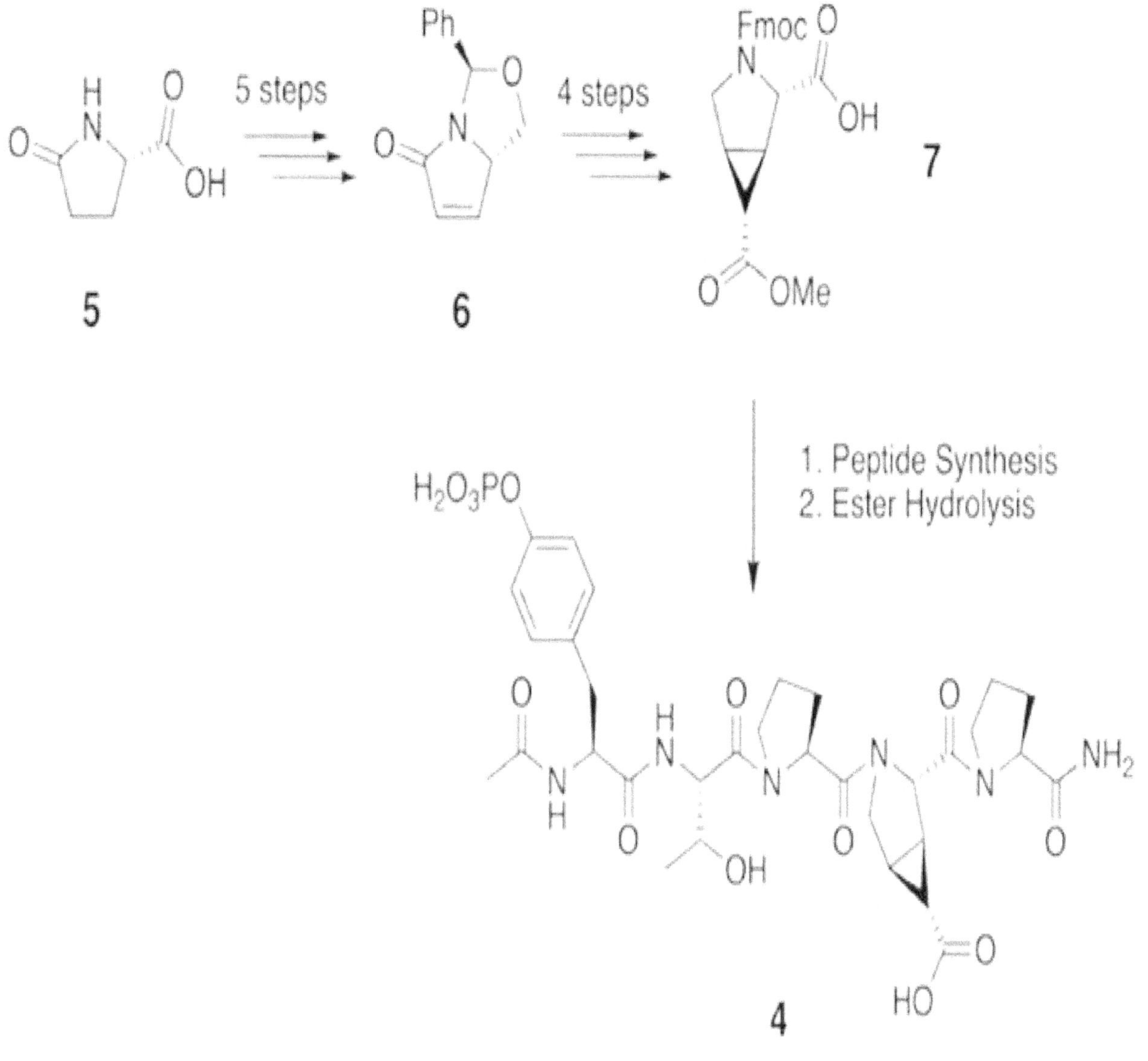

Fig10: some peptide substituted with unusual carboxyl surrogate residues.

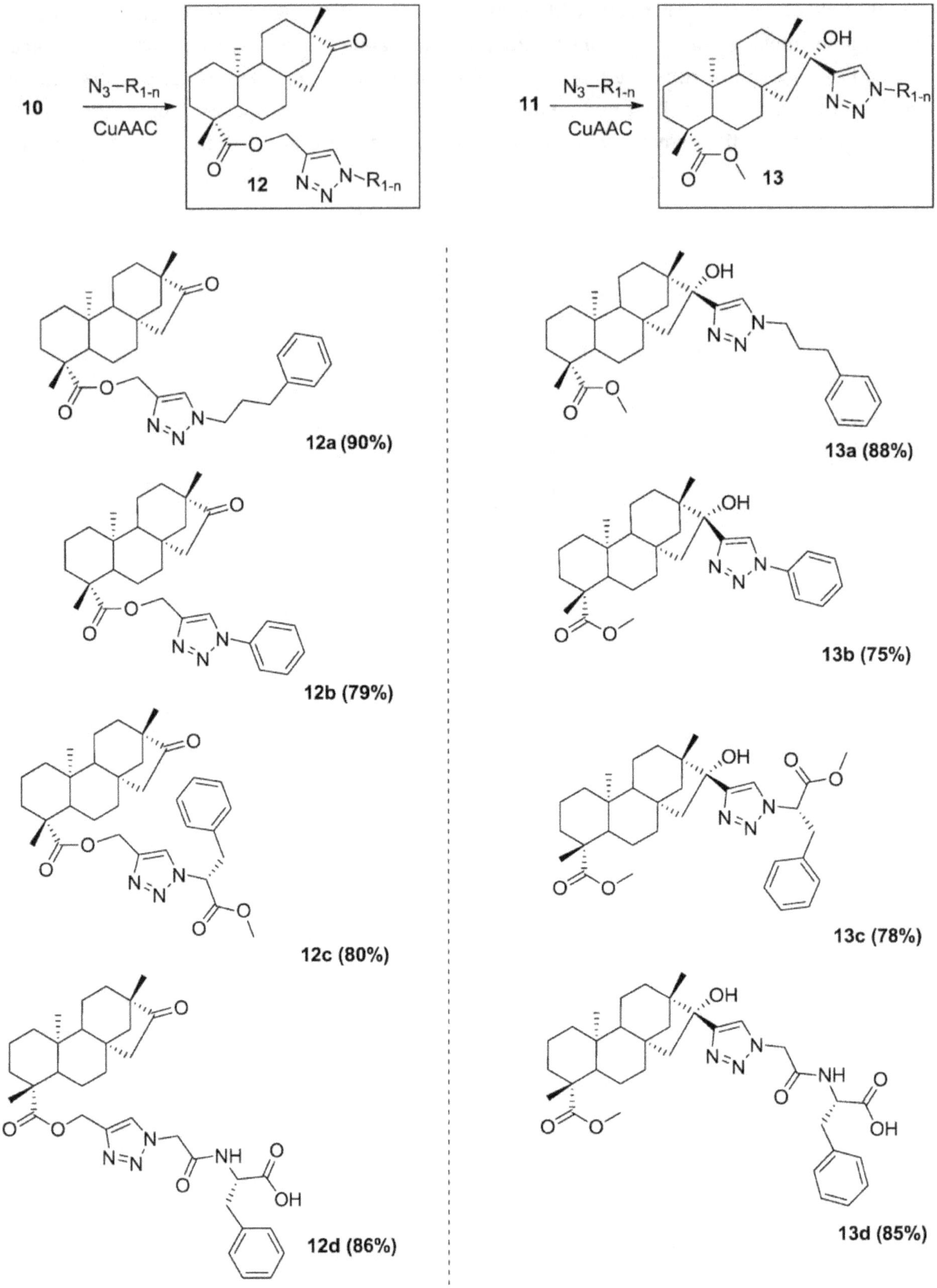

Fig11: structural examples of unusual surrogate residues.

The modification and revision of peptide libraries by the outcome of peptide reaction array with variable reagents to transume the components into new materials is an influential and prevailing resource of growing or intensifying the size and scope of the assortment. This is well regardedly known as "libraries from libraries" and the interesting fact is that this view of perception is not circumscribed only to peptides. For normal peptides filteration with varied alternatives comprises the synthesis of libraries of vinylogous amides, polycarbamates, assimilation of ureas and of a pepstatin residue. Here in these libraries the side chains schemes from each fourth instead of each third atom in the atomic chain so these are not nearly compacted representations to the amino acids. These peptides and pseudo peptide libraries have been substituted gradually by various assortments which contain small and more drug like molecules.

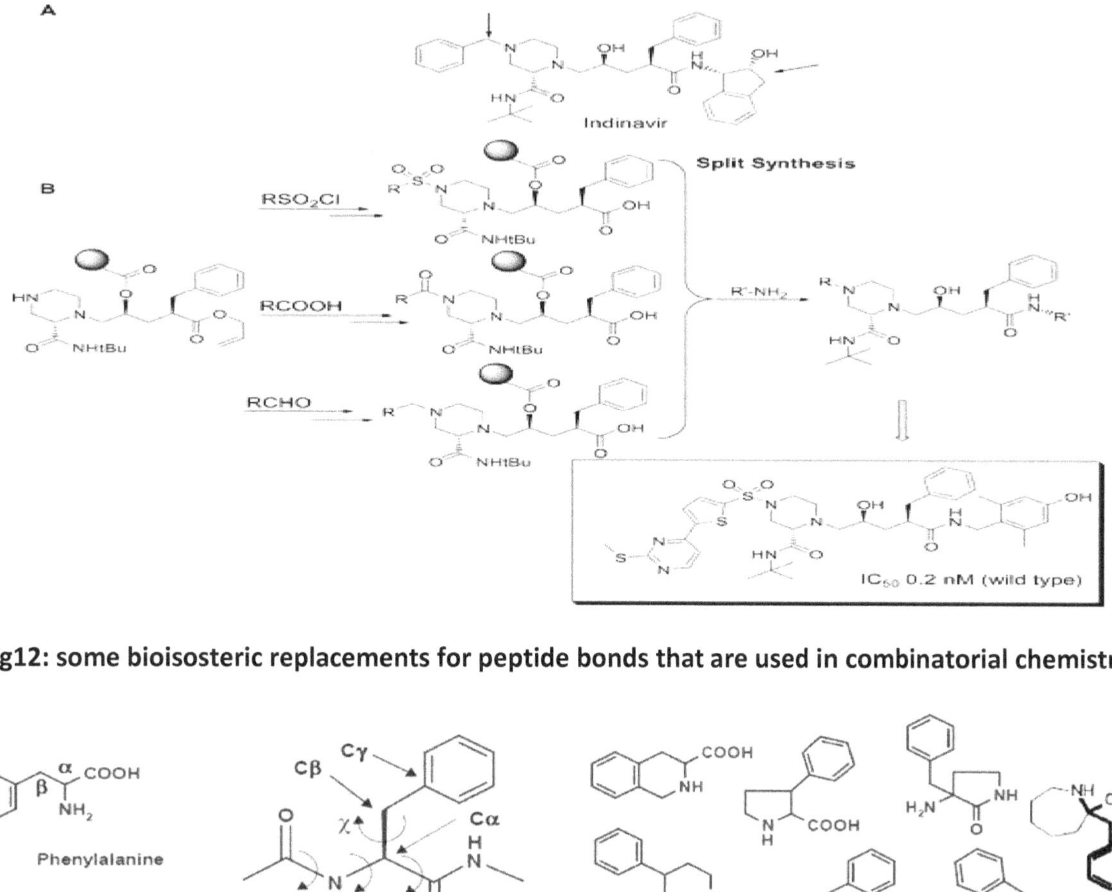

Fig12: some bioisosteric replacements for peptide bonds that are used in combinatorial chemistry.

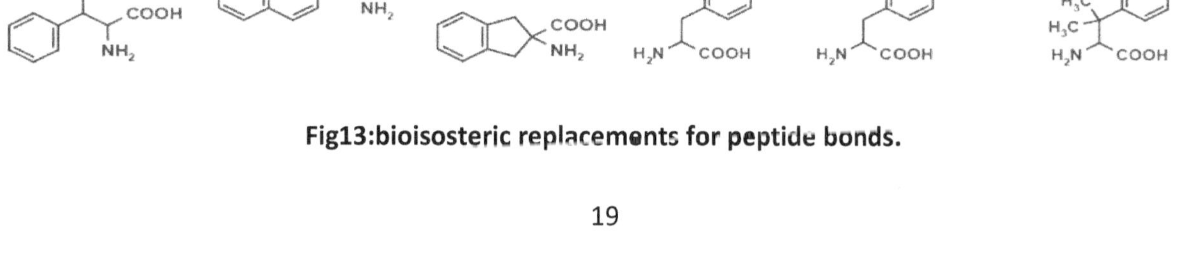

Fig13: bioisosteric replacements for peptide bonds.

The capability to make and test libraries which contain peptides and peptidomimetics of uncertain length with familiar primary structure numbering in the millions is well known and focussed and this is absolutely an enormous success.

Oligosaccharide arrays:

In most biological processes like cellular recognition and adhesion, cellular communication, immunology, carbohydrates play a very important role. This phenomenon alone is satisfactory to validate the construction of compound libraries. Very few chemically synthesised drugs have their place in the chemical lineage but the glycosides are not included here apparently decreasing few number of provocations. production and analysis of different kinds of oligosachharide libraries is far more problematic that producing peptides. The glycosidic linkages comprises of a stereogenic carbon and is comparetively difficult task to regulate or direct and the bonds are sensitive to acid and there are a lot of possibly opposing functional groups that can be point of attachment. If branching chains exists, their production is merely a vast method. The attraction of oligosachharides to their receptors are considerably less so by this assessment of lagre number of rigidly binding glycopeptides is much more communal. In spite of these obscuring issues such libraries are performing proogressively.

The primary and initial compund libraries of oligosachharides were moderately quite lesser, were usually not divided into single individual compounds and were not finely categorised. Chiefly in regard to their anomeric proportions. The reactants commonly comrised of defensive glycyl acceptors. The unprotected glycyl receptor libraries comprised of comparatively casual glycosidation products so remained impartially compound combinations which were almost extremely challenging to isolate. An influential libraryof this kind was that of Hindsgaul and his collegues which comprised of a combination of six alpha linked positional diglycoside isomers synthesised by solution phase chemistry. The instillation of a lipophilic anomeric ether on the glycyl acceptor moiety to enable the parting of the synthesised products is one of the most fascinating facts. The reactions were controlled on an additional basis at about 30% of its accomplishment permissible to diminish production of various glycosidation products.

In spite of such kinds of improvements and progressions, the suitable and appropriate programmed glycan production will persist to be tenuous. Novel developments has been introduced in chemical and engineering bulletin. Oligosachharide libraries can also be largely produced on beads as eemplified by 12-membered trisachharide library of Zhu and Boons and the 1300-membered mixture di- and tri- sachharide libraries of Kahne produced by the split and pool process with the use of halogen isotope prearranged beads for decoding.

The Kahne library was effectively analysed along with the mechanisms calmed devotedto the beads and the active beads were selected out by the pasture like technique.

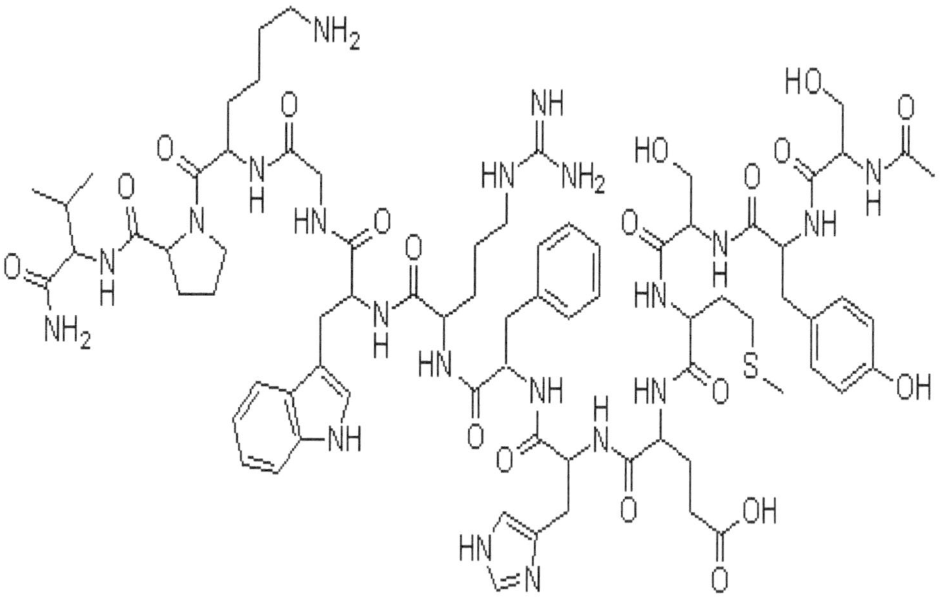

Ac-Ser-Tyr-Ser-Met-Glu-His-Phe-Arg-Trp-Gly-Lys-Pro-Val-NH₂

fig14: carbohydrate compound libraries illustrated with normal strings of hexones.

Nucleoside Arrays:

Normally there are five usually sustaining nucleic acid bases and two sugars. Therefore a completely comprehended compound library would be significantly lesser than those of peptides. The admiration of correspondants with synthetic bases or sugars magnifies or increases the potentials remarkably. Nucleoside building blocks and oligonucleotides themselves have achieved greater degree of focus on them by the asset of their essential biological outlines which comprises their application in antisense, antiviral and anticancer research. This conciousness of the significant therapeutic usefulness of nucleotide referents, intended to advance their strenght and avoid different biological and physical confines. Conventionally maximum nucleoside library creations eertions concerned derivatization of the nucleoside base constituent of priorly formed nucleosides. By the application of the above discussed policy both solution and solid phase synthesis, great numbers of nucleoside libraries have been build up.

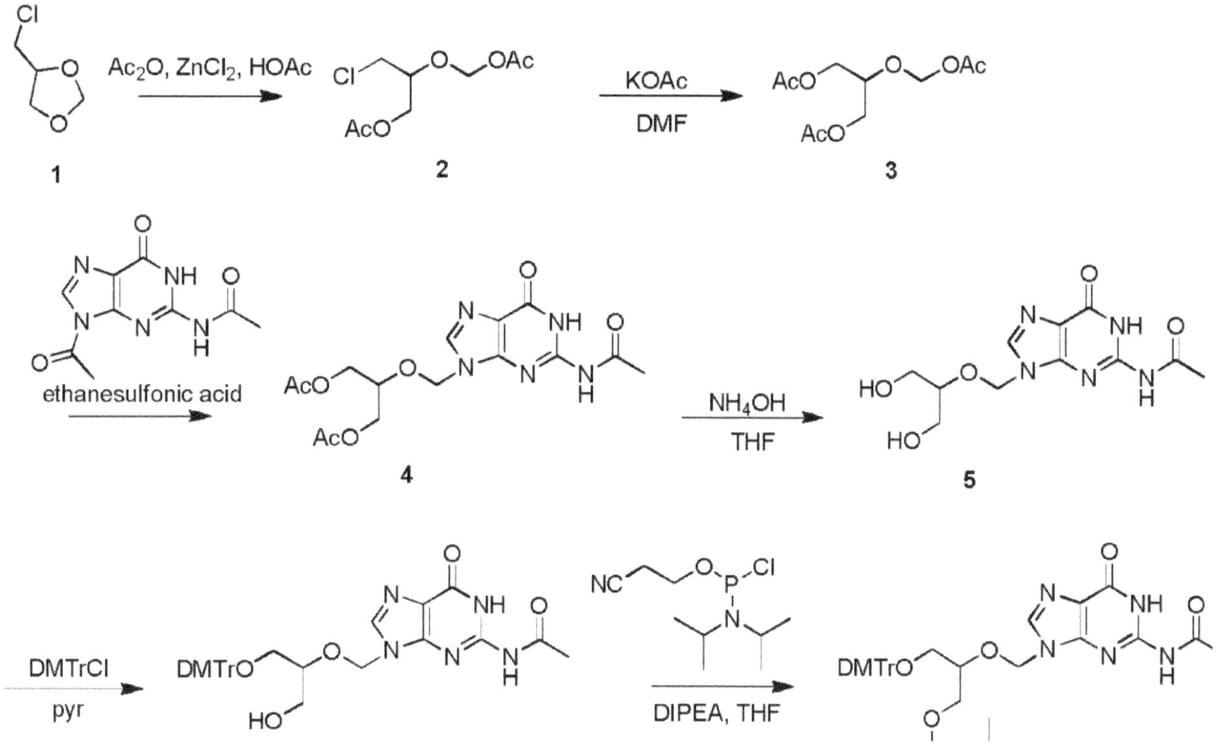

Fig15: Some examples of combinatorial synthesis of N2, N6- distributed diaminopurine nucleosides.

In a deliberately diverse solution phase method which includes microwave accelerated reaction of different unsynthetic and synthetic nucleobases or amines with an appropriately useful ribofuranosyl derivative under Vorbruggen condition directed to the speedy formulation of a physically varied nucleoside library. When analysed and associated to be equaled in standards to the glycosidation conditions, the application of microwave heating lead to a major valuable decrease in the reaction time. Extinguishing of the additional lewis acidic reagent along with triethanol amine in aqueous acetonitrile approved for direct high throughput MPLC purification f the nucleoside adduct which consists of reaction mixture. With the application of this method which is discussed above, a mixture of six varied acylated ribofuranosyl donors with a diversity of amine nucleophiles brought about the development of a library of greater than 400 nucleosides.

Lipid Arrays:

Lipid libraries have immensely been ignored. For saturated fatty acids, the development of carbon-carbon bonds and ester linkages is not problematic yet this concern of combinatorial chemistry is under improvement for its progression. Mixed triglycerides are sensibly comprehensible, chiefly initiating with oxiranemethanol to reslove the regioselectivity issues.

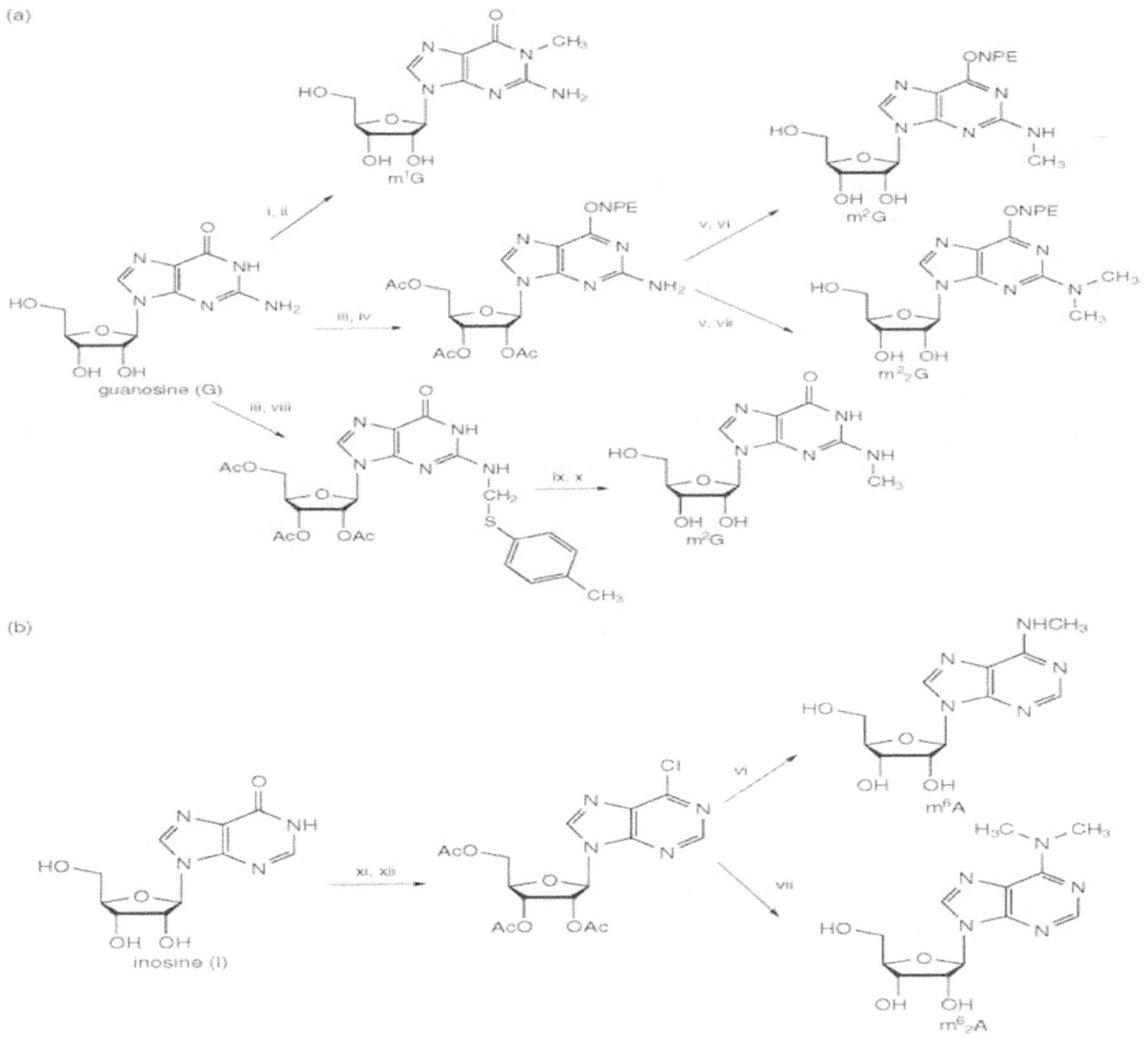

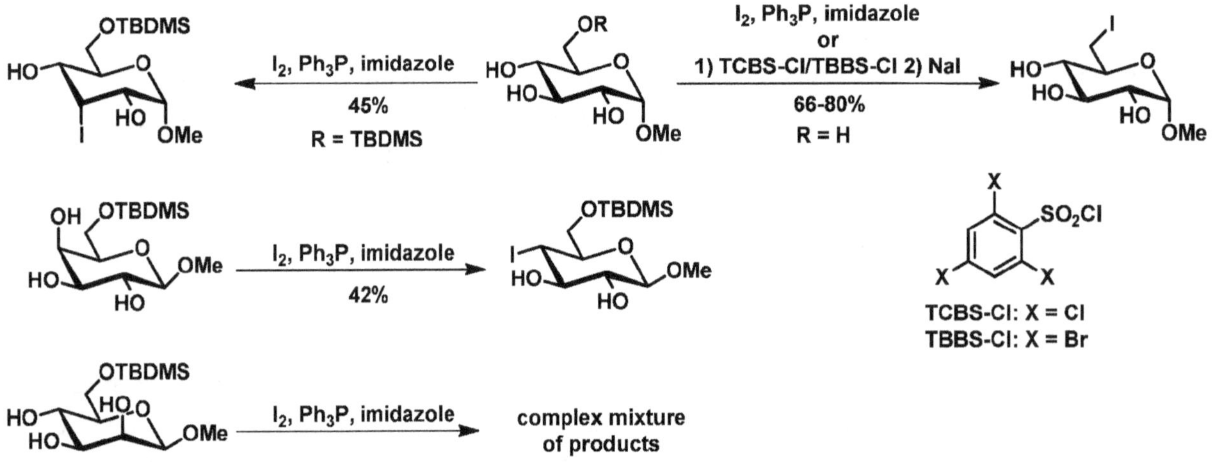

Fig16: Some examples of microwave assisted glycosidation approach to nucleoside libraries.

Steroids and different polyisoprenoids have been the centroids for cominatorial libraries. They are justly levelled molecules so have a reduced capability to scheme functional functional groups into three dimensional space. Yet they agonize from having efficacious molecular weights so less variety can be completed eith them with the purpose of attaining activity.

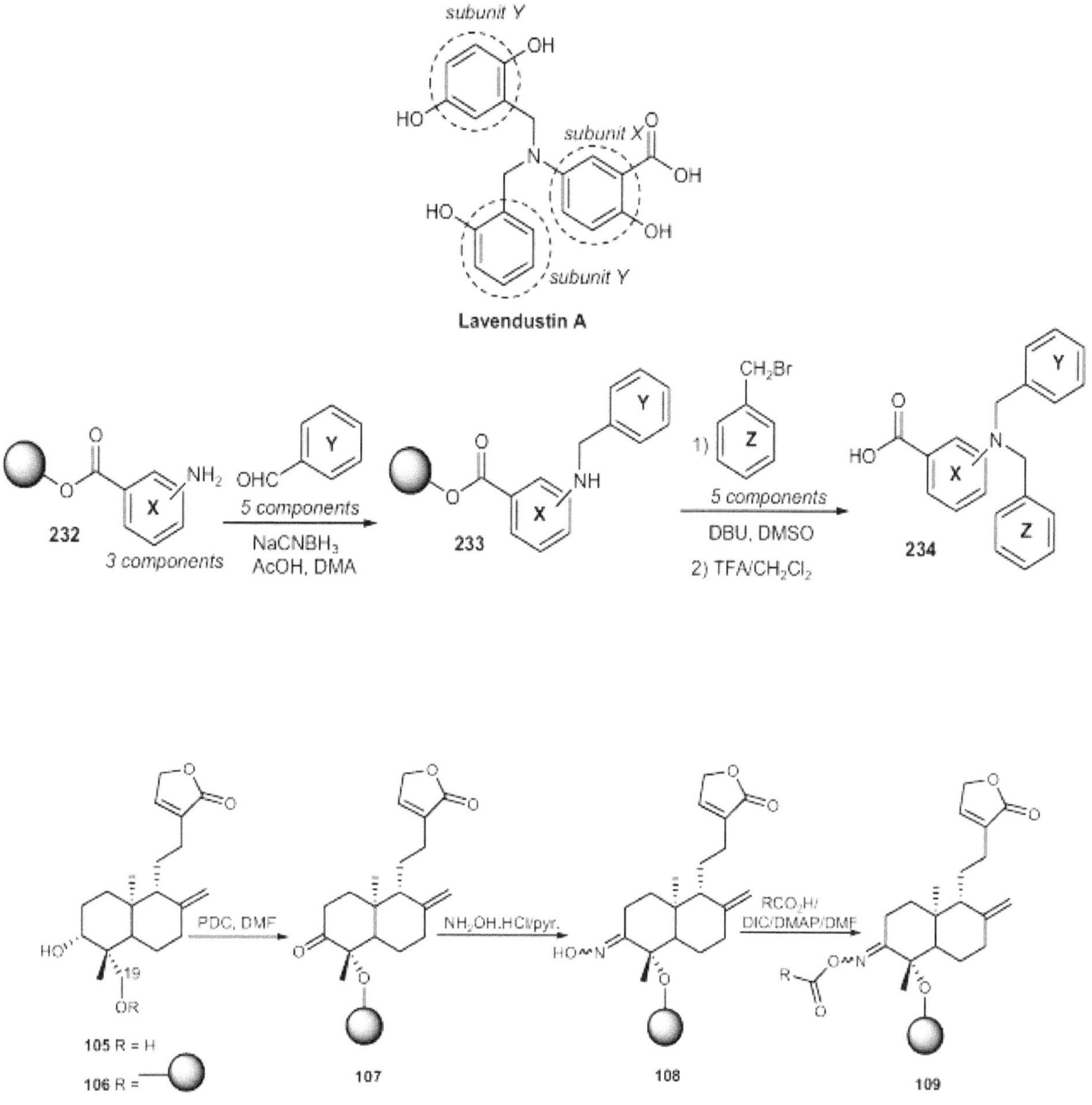

Fig17: Some examples of combinatorial library synthesis of chiral lipids.

References:

Mitscher LA, Dutta A. Combinatorial chemistry. In:Abraham D, editor. Burger's Medicinal chemistry. 6th ed., vol. 2. New Yor: john Wiley & Sons, Inc:2003. P 2-36.

Merrifeld RB solid phase peptide synthesis. I. The synthesis of a tetrapeptide. Jam chem soc 1963;85:2149-2154.

Bunin BA, Ellman JA.A general and expedient method for the solid-phase synthesis of 1,4-benzodiazepine derivatives. J Am Chem Soc 1992;114:10997-10998.

Weber A, von roedern E,Stilz HU. SynCar: an approach to automated synthesis J com chem 2005;7(2):178-84

Koppitz M, Eis K. Automated medical chemistry. Drug Discov Today 2006;11(11-12):561-568.

Koppitz M. Mazimizing efficiency in the production of compound libraries. J Comb Chem 2008;10(4):573-579.

Ojima I. Modern natural products chemistry and drug discovery. J med chem 2008;51(9):2587-2588.

Miertus S, Fassina G. Combinatorial chemistry. New Yor:pergamin: 1999.p 339

About The Author

During Pharmacy course I got a great opportunity to learn and explore things. I am very thankful to my staff that supported me in my work. The writer must believe that what she is doing the most valuable work for her- Afiya Ansari

www.ingramcontent.com/pod-product-compliance
Lightning Source LLC
Chambersburg PA
CBHW080533190526
45169CB00008B/3141